WHAT U NEED TO KNOW ABOUT CANCER?

WHAT U NEED
TO KNOW ABOUT
CANCER?

Jackie Young

XULON PRESS

Xulon Press
555 Winderley Pl, Suite 225
Maitland, FL 32751
407.339.4217
www.xulonpress.com

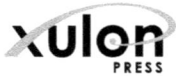

Xulon
PRESS

Paperback ISBN-13: 979-8-86850-273-6
Ebook ISBN-13: 979-8-86850-274-3

INTRODUCTION

ALTHOUGH CANCER IS SAID TO BE 100 OR EVEN 200 TYPES OF CANCER, THE TYPES DESCRIBED IN THIS BOOK ACCOUNT FOR NEARLY ALL THE CASES EACH CHAPTER IS DESIGNED TO PRESENT INFORMATION ON SPECIFIC TYPES OF CANCER. YOU MAY SEE MATERIAL REPEATED HOWEVER, THE DIAGNOSTIC TREATMENTS OR PROCEDURES MAY BE THE SAME. IT IS UNLIKELY THAT ANY ONE PERSON WILL WANT TO READ ABOUT EVERY TYPE OF CANCER TREATMENT THATS DISCUSSED IN THIS BOOK. PREVENTION AND EDUCATION THE KEYS TO GOOD HEALTH. WE NEED TO KNOW MORE ABOUT OURSELVES AND OUR OWN HEALTH. WHEN WE ARE WILLING TO EDUCATE OURSELVES ABOUT COMMON HEALTH DISORDERS AND DISEASES, THE WE CAN BE FULL PARTNERS IN OUR OWN HEALTHCARE. MY BOOK IS DESIGNED TO PROVIDE BASIC KNOWLEDGE THAT READERS WILL NEED IF THEY ARE TO TAKE SIGNIFICANT RESPONSIBILITY OF THEIR OWN HEALTH. THE INFORMATION IN MY BOOK IS NOT INTENDED TO REPLACE THE ADVICE OF YOUR DOCTOR. THIS BOOK IS TO INFORM AND EDUCATE THE READER WITH A VIEW TO MAKE THE PROPER CHOICES CONCERNING YOUR HEALTH. I ASSUME NO RESPONSIBILITY OR LIABILITY FOR THE DECISIONS AND JUDGEMENTS MADE AS A RESULT OF READING THIS BOOK. I HAVE 30 PLUS YEARS IN THE MEDICAL FIELD AND A MEDICAL RESEARCHER.

WHAT IS CANCER?

C ancer is the second leading cause of death in the United States. There are many types of cancer and not all of them behave the same or respond to the same treatment. Each form of cancer begins as a single cell, fertilized eggs begin dividing and for a while, there is just a ball of cells which all look the same, slowly the ball of cells begin to take on a human shape. In some places in the body, cells keep dividing and multiplying like for example, tiny fingers form and grow longer, in other places cells stop multiplying. A series of signals tells some cells to multiply and others to stop multiplying.

Cancer cells should not multiply, what should have been a single cell in the lining of your stomach becomes a growing ball of cells, this is called a primary tumor, first the ball of cancer cells pushes against and squashes the normal cells around it, then it starts to burrow through the normal cells this is called invasion. The invading cancer cells then reach blood vessel or lymph vessel and spread to other parts of the body. In a process called metastatic tumors every cell in the body has genes that if activated tell the cells to multiply and every cell has other genes that if activated tell the cell to stop multiplying, these genes are required for normal growth.

CANCER OF THE BLADDER

The bladder is a muscular balloon that stores and empties urine carried down from each of the two kidneys by a tube called a ureter. The bladder empties the urine through another tube which is the urethra, in women this is a very short tube in front of the vagina. In men the tube is a longer one that passes first through the prostate gland and along under the surface of the penis. Most bladder tumors look like mushrooms with stems attached to the inner lining of the bladder, these are called papillary tumors they are soft and crumbly and can be either benign or malignant. The other type of bladder cancer is called epidermoid carcinomas, this tumor grows directly on the lining of the bladder and tends to invade the muscular wall of the bladder.

SYMPTOMS

The first warning sign of bladder cancer is usually bloody urine, most of the time the blood appears suddenly, with little or no pain at all. Blood in the urine is not a sure sign that a person has bladder cancer. There could be other reasons for blood in the urine such as a urinary tract infection, a benign tumor or bladder stones. However, you might see blood one day and it disappears the next day, your urine may be clear for months. But with bladder cancer, sooner or later the blood will reappear, the amount is not related to the stage of the cancer. Sometimes the bleeding can cause discomfort, as well as blood clots causing painful muscle spasms in the bladder.

DIAGNOSIS

To determine whether your symptoms are caused by bladder cancer or some other condition, samples of your urine are examined with a microscope it is possible to see cancer cells in the urine if they are present. The doctor may decide that you should have an x-ray called an intravenous pyelogram. For the pyelogram test a special dye is injected into the bloodstream during the injection, you may have a warm feeling, this is usually the only reaction you will have. The dye passes into the urine in the bladder this makes the bladder more visible in the x-ray pictures. The doctor can recognize any abnormality on the outline of the bladder. To find out the exact size and location of the tumor, the doctor uses an instrument called a cystoscope, this allows him to see inside the bladder the cystoscope is inserted through the urethra into the bladder. If a suspicious area is seen during the test a small sample of tissue will be taken. Examination of the tissue is the only sure way of finding out whether it is cancer or not. If a tumor is large the doctor may be able to feel it through the rectum or vagina with his fingers. However, a biopsy is still necessary to determine if its cancer or not.

TREATMENT

Your treatment must be tailored to your individual needs, your doctor will consider a number of factors in determining the best treatment for you. The doctor may remove a single papillary tumor using a cystoscope. When several tumors are found, the treatment generally is to remove the tumors and surrounding tissue by surgery. After surgery a solution that contains an anticancer drug may be instilled into the bladder to decrease the chance of the tumor recurring. If your doctor does not consider surgery is advisable, radiation therapy may be used. Cancer of the bladder seldom requires the removal of the bladder. If the cancer has started to spread out of the bladder, the surgeon can often stop it by removing other nearby organs, in women the organs may be the ovaries, fallopian tubes, the uterus and the portion of the vagina that contains the urethra. In men the prostate gland, seminal vesicles and in some cases the urethra. If all the cancer cannot be removed by surgery or destroyed by radiation and chemotherapy, treatment with anticancer drugs can be administered.

BONE CANCER

The 206 bones in your body serve several purposes, your bones support and protect internal organs, for example, the ribs protect the lungs, the skull protects the brain, etc. the muscles pull against the bones to make the body move. The bone marrow in your body makes and stores blood cells, it is the soft spongy tissue in the center of many bones. Cancer that begins in the bone is called bone cancer it is most often found in the arms and legs. However, bone cancer can occur in any bone in the body. Primary bone cancers are called Sarcomas there are several types of Sarcomas, each type begins in a different kind of bone tissue, the most common are Osteosarcoma, Ewing and Chondrosarcoma. Osteosarcoma is the most common type of bone cancer in young people, it usually occurs between ages 10 and 25, males are affected more often than females, this type of cancer usually starts in the ends of bone, where new tissue forms as a young person grows, it usually affects the long bones of the arms or legs. Ewing's Sarcoma affects teenagers most often, it forms in the middle part of long bones in the thigh and upper arm, it also occurs in the ribs. Chondrosarcoma is found mainly in adults, this type of tumor forms in cartilage, which is the rubbery tissue around joints. Other types of bone cancer include Fibrosarcoma, malignant giant cell tumor and Chordoma.

These rare cancers are most seen in people over 30, bone cancers are quite rare. However, it is not unusual for cancer to spread to the bones from other parts of the body, when this happens the disease is not called bone cancer, each type of cancer is named for the organ or the tissue where it begins.

Symptoms

Symptoms of bone cancer tends to develop slowly, depending on the type, location and size of the tumor, pain is the most frequent symptom. Sometimes a firm slightly tender lump on the bone can be felt through the skin. In some cases, bone cancer interferes with normal movement, and can cause bones to break. However, these signs of cancer could be caused by other serious problems, only your doctor can tell for sure.

How is bone cancer diagnosed?

The doctor usually orders x-rays and blood tests, x-rays can show the location, shape and size of the bone tumor, a biopsy is the only way to tell whether cancer is present. Treatment This disease is usually treated with surgery, radiation therapy or chemo therapy the doctor often uses a combination of treatment methods depending on the patient needs.

CANCER OF THE BRAIN

There are two types of cancerous brain tumors primary and secondary. Primary brain tumors start in brain tissue, secondary brain tumors are are cancers that starts in another organ, most commonly the lung or breast, and spread to the brain. Secondary brain tumors are more common than primary tumors and occur in 25% of people who have cancer elsewhere in the body, brain tumors can affect both genders and can occur at any age. Secondary tumors are more common later in life when all cancers are more likely to develop. Symptoms Some brain tumors are discovered when they are still small and cause a seizure or hemorrhage most brain tumors produce no symptoms until they grow large enough to compress neighboring brain tissue and can cause an impairment such as weakness of the arm or leg and may cause difficulty speaking sometime a headache is the only symptom of a brain tumor. A headache in someone who usually does not have headaches may be the first symptom some rare occasions an unexplained personality change may happen.

TREATMENT OPTIONS

If a tumor goes untreated it can lead to permanent brain damage most types are fatal despite the best treatment, early discovery for benign and some malignant tumors early, offer the best chance of recovery. To look for a brain tumor, a number of tests including {cat scan, a {MRI} to determine the size as well as the location of any tumors since secondary brain tumors develop from other cancers in other organs the doctor will order radiology tests also of other parts of your body if surgery is needed a cerebral angiography may also be required to further evaluate the size as well as the site of the tumor depending on what the doctor finds, you might be referred to see a neurosurgeon, neurologist or a oncologist. Surgery to remove some benign and malignant tumors can be successful, however depending if the tumor cannot be cut out because it is attached to vital brain structures, recurrence is likely, if the tumor cannot be completely removed or is incurable, it is sometimes possible to remove a portion of it in order to reduce pressure and relieve symptoms radiation therapy or chemotherapy may be used as well as corticosteroid drugs may be given to reduce the swelling of brain tissue and some anti-convulsant drugs can control seizures related to the tumor growth. BREAST CANCER Breast cancer is the most common cancer in women, like all cancers, it begins in one spot and grows larger for months or years. Breast cancer can metastasize (spread) to other parts of the body through the lymphatic system and the blood stream.

RISK FACTORS

Breast cancer results from changing in the genes of breast cells. The precise causes of these genetic mutations are not fully understood. Nevertheless, age is the most significant risk factor for breast cancer. Breast cancer is uncommon in women younger than 35, the risk is higher in women over 50 and especially in women over 60. The risk of developing breast cancer at 60 is about 26 times greater than at 35. Other factors that play into breast cancer are health history, family history, age and estrogen levels.

CERVICAL CANCER

An estimated 15,000 American women will develop invasive cervical cancer this year, an estimated 8,500 women will die of this disease. Cervical cancer has increased in recent years in women.

DYSPLASIA AND CANCER OF THE CERVIX

Dysplasia is the presence of abnormal cells. Dysplasia is classified as mild, moderate, or severe, it often develops in women between the age of 25 and 35. However, it may develop in women in their teens or early twenties, it rarely causes symptoms and can be detected only by an exam that includes a pap smear. Dysplasia does not always go on to develop into cancer, some women it go through a series of changes that then develops into cancer If it not treated. Almost 100% of cases early detected is curable if treatment is started at the time of diagnosis. If left untreated it can advance to invasive cancer. Invasive cancer mainly occurs between the ages of forty and sixty.

SYMPTOMS

Symptoms most often include abnormal bleeding from the vagina. The bleeding may be particularly noticeable after intercourse, other forms of abnormal bleeding includes spotting between menstrual periods and after douching and bleeding after menopause. If any of these symptoms develops consult your doctor immediately. The sooner invasive cancer is diagnosed and treated the better the chances are for cure, if left untreated it will continue to grow and eventually may spread beyond the cervix to other parts of the body.

WOMEN AT RISK

Some women are more likely than others to develop abnormal cervical cells. Women at risk include women who began having sexual intercourse with numerous male partners, women who began sexual intercourse before age eighteen. Virgins almost never develop cervical cancer, but all women who sexually active have some risk of this disease.

DIAGNOSIS

Your doctor will perform a pap smear test where samples of cells are collected from the cervix and cervical canal. This procedure is painless and quick. To get an accurate test do not douche during the 24 hours before your exam. The medical laboratory determines whether the cells appear normal or abnormal and if abnormal to what degree. The laboratory report is sent to your doctor. Your pelvic exam should include inspection of your external genitals, cervix and vagina in addition the doctor should exam your breast for unusual lumps at every exam while teaching you how to check your breast each month. Your doctor can look directly at your cervix and vagina during your pelvic exam if any areas on your cervix or vagina looks abnormal your doctor may remove a tiny amount of tissue for microscopic examination, this is called a biopsy. The biopsy procedure may be uncomfortable, or in some cases slightly painful, bleeding after your biopsy is common. An abnormal pap smear test or biopsy results is not proof that you have precancerous or cancerous a condition, however it means you will need other diagnostic test done. Tests causing little discomfort that your doctor c I cannot perform in the office is a test where iodine solution is applied to your cervix called a schiller's test, followed by biopsy of abnormal areas. Colposcopic- an instrument that magnifies the surface of the cervix and vagina, may be used to pinpoint change my mindset which I'm still struggling we still working on it go take every course then you will be notified Saturday schools suspicious areas for biopsy. Your doctor may also want to scrape small amounts of tissue that lines your cervical canal. If your doctor decides it's advisable to take some tissue scrapings of the cervical and the lining of the uterus, this is called a DNC or to remove tissue from the cervix and cervical canal is called [conization or cone biopsy}

TREATMENT

Surgery for invasive cancer of the cervix involves removal of the uterus, cervix, upper vagina and some surrounding tissue, plus removal of the lymph nodes in the area which is called a radical hysterectomy. Radiation therapy may be used, both internal and external are often used. Internal radiation therapy requires a brief hospitalization. Radioactive material such as radium is inserted into the uterus and vagina for a short period of time. When chemotherapy is prescribed, the anticancer drugs are often injected into the bloodstream.

CANCER OF THE COLON AND RECTUM

The lowest part of the digestive tract is the colon, also called the large bowel, it is the last 5 to 6 feet of the intestine the last 5 to 6 inches of the colon is the rectum. After food is digested, the solid food passes through the colon and rectum to the anus where it is passed out of the body. When illness affects the colon or rectum, a number of symptoms may appear.

Warning signs of possible problems:

Diarrhea or constipation, blood in the stool (either bright red or very dark stools) that are smaller in width than usual, stomach discomfort, bloating fullness, cramps, frequent gas pains, a feeling that the bowels not emptying completely, loss of weight and constant tiredness. These symptoms may be caused by a number of problems such as ulcers, or an inflamed colon.

Diagnosis of colorectal cancer:

The doctor usually performs some specific examinations to check the rectal area, the doctor inserts a glove, finger into the rectum and gently feels for any bumps. The doctor may also perform a test called a procto to look at the rectum and colon, for this exam a hollow, lighted instrument called a sigmoidoscope is inserted into the anus. About 60 percent of colon and rectal cancers can be found with the procto exam. To find out whether there is blood in the stool, a stool sample (a smear) is placed on special a slide to be examined by the lab. Another test that might also may be given is {lower g.i. series} x –ray pictures of the colon that are taken after a thick solution of barium flows into the bowel through an enema tube. The barium shows an outline of the large intestine and may reveal tumors that were not found in the other tests. If there is a need to look further, the doctor can see the entire length of the colon through a thin, lighted flexible tube called a colonoscope. If an abnormal growth is found, the doctor will need to remove a small sample for a biopsy. If a malignant tumor is found, the doctor will want to start a treatment plan designed to fit the type and the extent of the cancer.

<u>TREATMENT</u>

There are three basic ways to treat cancer of the colon and rectum, surgery, x-ray therapy and drug therapy, this is the standard treatment for most colon and rectal cancers. If surgery is recommended it will depend on the location and the size of the cancerous tumor. The surgeon may be able to remove only the part of the bowel where the cancer is and rejoin the healthy section all at once. This operation is called a bowel resection, it is usually all that is required. If the cancer is in the right side of the colon or in the long section across the top (the transverse colon) the cancer is blocking the bowel, a procedure called a (colostomy) a colostomy can be temporary or permanent. In both cases the surgeon removes the cancerous section of the bowel and create an opening in the abdomen, this is called a stoma so that waste is routed out of the body without passing through the lower colon and rectum. A temporary colostomy is done to allow the lower colon and rectum to rest and heal, especially if the cancer is close to the rectum. When the patient has healed enough, a second operation is done to close the stoma in order for the body to resume to it's normal digestive tract functions. Sometimes if the cancer is in the lower rectum, the rectum is removed and a permanent colostomy is needed. Rectal cancers that are found early sometimes can be treated without removal of the entire rectum. About 85 percent of patients with colon or rectal cancers do not require a permanent colostomy. A permanent colostomy is a reusable bag that's attached to a stoma to collect waste matter. it is worn continually but it does show under your clothing. A enterostomal therapist will teach the patient how to take care of it, the treatment required for some patients, will also include removal of the lymph nodes. There is a chance the cancer will spread to new areas. Radiation therapy may be used before surgery to shrink the tumor, or after surgery to destroy any cancer cells that were not removed in the operation. Radiation therapy may relieve the pain that some cancers cause. There are certain known factors, that increase a person's risk of developing colorectal cancer. This type of cancer is seen more often in people over 40, it is seldom seen in a younger person. {I.} a person who has close relatives with an in inherited condition known as familial polyposis, has a much greater chance of developing colorectal cancer. people with familial polyposis develop a large number of polyps in the intestines and polyps in the mucus membrane often become cancerous. an estimated 135,000

Americans are diagnosed and 56,000 die of colorectal cancer each year, making it the second leading cause of cancer related death.

CANCER OF THE ESOPHAGUS

The esophagus is the muscular tube that carries food from the throat to the stomach.in adults, the esophagus is about 10 inches long. Cancer of the esophagus is a disease of the body's cells, like all cancer, your cells are tiny structures that make up parts of the body, your skin, your heart, lungs, and bones. Although cells of various organs are different in shape and how they function, all cells reproduce themselves by dividing when cells division is not orderly and controlled, the abnormal growth occurs into masses of tissue called tumors buildup. These tumors can be benign or malignant. Benign tumors do not spread, they can usually be removed completely and are not likely to reoccur. However, malignant tumors called cancers invade neighboring tissues and organs and can spread to other parts of the body, forming new growth, this called metastases, even if the main tumor is removed, the cancer reoccurs because cancer cells have spread.

SYMPTOMS

The most common symptom of esophageal cancer is difficulty in swallowing, there could be a feeling that swallowed food is sticking along the way to the stomach. Most of the time meat is usually the first food to cause this sticking sensation. This feeling can occur whether food is stuck and blocking the esophagus. Pain can also be a symptom, it may be a momentary burning as food is swallowed, and pain may also come from behind the breastbone.

DIAGNOSIS

To determine whether your symptoms are caused by esophageal cancer or some other condition, the doctor may order an x-ray where you will be asked to swallow a liquid containing barium sulfate, which is a substance that makes parts of your body more visible in x ray pictures, using an x-ray machine called a fluoroscope, the doctor can watch the motion of the esophagus as the barium flows down toward your stomach, also regular x-ray pictures maybe taken when the esophagus is completely coated by the barium. The doctor can recognize an abnormality in the outline of the esophagus seen on the fluoroscope along with the x-ray pictures, if abnormal areas are seen, the doctor can use a slender instrument called an esophagoscope to examine them more closely. The doctor will apply an anesthetic to the throat to numb the area. The instrument is passed through the mouth and throat into the esophagus, the esophagoscope allows the doctor to see the suspected area and to remove a small sample of the tissue when the tissue is placed under a microscope it will reveal whether it is cancerous or benign. The removal of the tissue and microscopic examination is called a biopsy. If no abnormal growth is seen, the esophagus may be washed with a solution inserted and removed through the esophagoscope, the solution is then examined for cancer cells. If cancer is diagnosed usually it's best to begin your treatment in a hospital where there is expert staff and resources to begin effective treatment. Before your treatment you might want to get a second opinion to confirm your diagnosis.

TREATMENT

Radiation therapy is the method most often used to treat esophageal cancer, in some cases, surgery might be performed to remove all of the cancer, this opportunity is usually better when the cancer is limited to the lower part of the esophagus. Radiation therapy is sometimes is either used before or after surgery

CANCER OF THE GALLBLADDER AND BILE DUCT

Cancerous tumors of the gallbladder and bile ducts are rare, people with gallstones are at a slightly higher risk there may not be any symptoms at first, there may be some tenderness in the upper right portion of the abdomen, also jaundice (yellowing of the whites of the eyes and skin) itchy skin and weight loss. If the doctor believes there is cancer, he or she will order an ultrasound, if the cancer has not spread the gallbladder and bile duct may be removed if the cancer has spread to the liver or other organs survival rates are less likely.

CARCINOID TUMORS

Carcinoid tumors are a rare type of cancer that mostly forms in the appendix, intestine or lungs. The tumors release large quantities of the hormone called serotonin along with other active substances, also there are no symptoms unless the tumors spread, in case it has spread, the serotonin which is released into the bloodstream may cause recurring diarrhea along with abdominal cramps, wheezing and puffy eyes. Some carcinoid tumors that spread are fatal, there are also rare forms that do not release hormones and are usually not a problem. The doctor may order blood and urine tests to confirm, also an ultrasound or ct scan to verify the presence of tumors. If the tumors are diagnosed early, they can be surgically removed. Chemotherapy can also help reduce the size of tumors.

CANCER OF THE KIDNEYS

The kidneys are a matched pair of vital organs located below your liver and stomach and near your backbone on either side, shaped like a kidney bean, with a slight indentation on one side. The adult kidney is 4 to 5 inches long and 2 to 3 inches wide and weighs about a half a pound. The kidneys helps removes waste from the body by making urine, they do this by filtering urea, salt and other substances from the blood as it flows through the kidneys. There are three tubes that enter each kidney at the point of indentation, the renal vein, the renal artery and the ureter, the long tube down which the urine flows to the bladder. The shell enclosing the kidney is called the capsule, inside the kidney the blood is filtered by thousands of filament-like renal tubules. The renal pelvis collects urine and funnels it into the ureter. The kidneys glands also manufacture and secrete a variety of hormones. Cancer of the kidney, like other cancers, is a disease of the body's cells of your body such as your bones, skin and heart.

Kidney cancer is a malignant growth of kidney tissue generally kidney cancers spread to other parts less quickly than some other cancers. Kidney cancer is usually difficult to identify early because it does not cause symptoms in the early stages. A cancerous tumor of the kidney does not usually interfere with kidney function until it is large, usually between 60% and 75% of patients treated in the early stage of kidney survive. Renal cell carcinomas accounts for about 75% of all kidney cancers, men are affected twice as often as women. Usually men over 50 risk for having this type of cancer increases if you have been exposed to asbestos, cadmium or gasoline and if a relative has had this type of cancer. Transitional cell cancer the same of cancer that affects the bladder, can also be located in a ureter of the kidney, this kind occurs more often in people who has used painkillers containing phenacetin for a long time. wilms tumors is another type of kidney cancer that occurs most often in children.

<u>SYMPTONS</u>

The most common symptom of kidney cancer is visible blood in the urine. The blood may be present one day and not seen the next day, blood in the urine can be a sign of a number of disorders other than cancer, but no matter what the cause is you should see your doctor. Other common symptoms of kidney cancer is the presence of a lump or mass in the abdomen and pain in the side, like all cancers kidney cancer can cause fatigue and loss of appetite. TYPES OF ADULT KIDNEY CANCERS More than 8 out of 10 kidney cancers are called renal carcinomas sometimes called renal cell carcinomas is most likely to occur in adults.

TREATMENT OPTIONS

See your doctor if you have blood in your urine. if cancer is suspected the doctor may order imaging tests such as x-rays of the kidneys, ureters and bladder, also an MRI and a cat scan of your kidney may be included as well as a bone scan or chest x-ray may be performed to make sure the cancer has nor spread. Renal cell carcinoma is usually treated by removing the diseased kidney, when the tumor is small (you can function with one kidney) if a person has transitional cell cancer, the most common treatment is to remove the kidney along with the ureter and part of the bladder.

CANCER OF THE LARYNX

The larynx, or voice box is composed of the epiglottis, false cords and true cords. the air you breathe enters the nose or mouth, from there it goes through the oropharynx, the epiglottis and into the trachea and into the lungs. The epiglottis closes during swallowing and prevents food from entering the larynx. The true vocal cords produces sound, when air passes through the larynx it causes the vocal cords to vibrate.

SYMPTONS

One of the most common symptoms of laryngeal cancer is a prolonged hoarseness. Any hoarseness lasting for more than three weeks should be reported to your doctor, hoarseness associated with cancer of the larynx is often caused by cancer originating on the vocal cords, but cancer may occur elsewhere in the larynx, either above or below the vocal cords and cause symptoms such as change in voice pitch, lump in the throat, coughing, pain in breathing or swallowing, or even ear ache. in some cases, hoarseness may not develop until much later or if at all.

DIAGNOSIS

The doctor will examine your larynx using a laryngeal mirror, which looks like a dentist's mirror with a long handle. Doctors can detect most tumors of the larynx by using this mirror, in addition, a thorough examination of the lymph nodes in the neck also is important. The doctor can examine your lymph nodes by feeling them or x-ray and fluoroscopic test can also help the doctor to determine the actual size, extent and the effect of the tumor.

Also, the exact site of the primary tumor and any evidence that the tumor may have spread, it is very important to the scheduling the appropriate treatment. If the doctor finds a tumor or other evidence of an unusual growth a biopsy will be arranged to determine whether it is benign or malignant.

TREATMENT

Most doctors agree that radiation therapy is probably the best treatment for early localized laryngeal cancer and successful radiation therapy often produces minimum after effects. Surgery or a combination of surgery is generally used for larger laryngeal cancer.

If the doctor determines that your larynx must be removed, a surgical operation called a total laryngectomy is performed or a partial laryngectomy may be needed leaving a normal or slightly hoarse voice. After the larynx is removed, the pharynx is closed so that food can be swallowed normally. The upper trachea is sutured to an opening in the skin so that air can pass through (this procedure is called a tracheostomy) and enter the lungs, after the operation the patient will breathe through this stoma, rather than breathing through the nose and mouth. If the cancer has spread to other tissues in the neck, then a more extensive operation called a neck dissection will be performed at the same time of the laryngectomy. A neck dissection is the surgical removal of the lymph nodes and surrounding structure within the neck. When cancer of the larynx spreads it usually goes to the tissue in the neck first rather than other parts of the body. If a laryngectomy is the necessary form of treatment, the patient can learn to speak again through a technique known as esophageal speech this substituted speech is produced by expelling swallowed air from the esophagus. This method is best learned from a qualified speech therapist.

CANCER OF THE LIVER

Cancers that have started in other organs such as the gastrointestinal tract, breast and the lungs often spread to the liver, where they start to grow. The liver is very vulnerable to metastatic cancer because of its large size and the large amount of blood that flows through it. Cancer that originates in the liver is called primary liver-cancer. There are two types of primary liver cancer, hematoma and cholangiocarcinoma. Hematoma develops in the liver cells and is more common in men who has long term liver disease such as hepatitis and cirrhosis and who are older than 50. Cholangiocarcinoma develops in the bile duct and tends to affect young adults it is more common in people with ulcerative colitis. In the early stages, liver cancer will often cause no symptoms. Pain in the upper right portion of the abdomen is usually the first specific symptom, along with fatigue, weight loss and the loss of appetite. Jaundice (the yellowing of the white of the eyes and skin) and the development of swelling of the abdomen are symptoms of more advanced disease.

TREATMENT OPTIONS

If the doctor is suspicious of liver cancer test are performed to examine the liver such as ultrasound, computed tomography (cat scan) mri (magnetic resonance imaging) as well as magnetic resonance angiography of the hepatic artery and a liver biopsy. The doctor will also do a blood test to see how well the liver is functioning and to look for proteins that are made by primary liver cancers, or by cancers that start in the large intestine and often spread to the liver. To determine the stage of the cancer laparoscopic or conventional surgery may be performed to see how far the cancer has spread. With primary liver tumors that have not yet spread outside the liver, is sometimes possible for surgery to remove all of the tumor with primary liver tumors, and nearly always with secondary liver tumors surgical removal of the tumor is performed only when the tumor is blocking a vital structure such as a bile duct. Chemotherapy can be injected through a catheter directly into the artery that provides the blood supply to the tumor, in this way higher concentrations of the toxic medicine can be applied to the tumor. Radiation and other newer procedures are also available to reduce pain.

ORAL CANCER

Each year approximately 43,250 people are newly diagnosed with oral cancer in the United States alone, oral cancer is one the largest group of cancers which fall into the head and neck group. Other cancers in the head and neck group is from treatment and they are at their lowest the thyroid and larynx cancers, they are not included in the number. About 43% of people diagnosed with oral cancer will not survive no longer than five years. The death rate from oral cancer is very high. The high death rate is directly related to two factors, the first is to be aware, knowing that the lifestyle choices you make such as tobacco use and other risks are causes of this disease. Knowing the risk factors greatly reduces your chance of developing this disease. Early detection is the second factor that will reduce your risk, most oral cancers can be caught early. With early detection, survival rates are high. Oral cancer screenings are effective ways of finding cancer at its early stage and is highly curable, these screenings are painless, quick as well as inexpensive.

RISK FACTORS YOU CAN CONTROL

- Tobacco use

- Excessive alcohol consumption

- The combined use of tobacco and alcohol

- Excessive unprotected exposure to sun

- Low intake of vegetables and fruits

- HPV 16 a viral infection

An increasing numbers of young people, who are non-smokers are being diagnosed with oral cancer. Persistent HPV 16 viral infection is the same virus that is responsible for 95% of all cervical cancer, individuals carrying this virus are not likely to know that they have it. There are no outwards symptoms. there are no preventative measures that will prevent sexual transmission of the virus. In adults limiting the number of sexual partners decreases your risk of contracting the virus. Older adults tend to develop more diseases in general, including oral cancer as their immune system is less efficient. However, the HPV disease can happen at any age. Statistics show males get oral cancer more often than females. The HPV virus impacts men more than women.

SIGNS AND SYMPTOMS

In the early stages of oral cancers development is often painless, physical signs may not be obvious, that is why this is a very dangerous disease. Regular screenings having knowledge about oral cancer and its symptoms will be very helpful in discovering tissue changes, when cure and survival are most likely. EARLY INDICATORS Discolorations of the soft tissue of the mouth, usually red or white. Any sore that does not heal within 14 days. Any hoarseness which last for a prolonged time.

ADVANCED SYMPTOMS

A sensation that something is stuck in your throat. numbness in in the oral region, difficulty in in swallowing, ear pain that sometimes occur on one side only, a lump or thickening which develops in the mouth or on the neck, difficulty in moving the muscles of the mouth, lips and tongue.

CANCER OF THE PANCREAS

The pancreas is a spongy, tube-shaped organ about 6 inches long. It is located in the back of the abdomen, behind the stomach. The head of the pancreas is on the right side of the abdomen, it is con-nected to the duodenum, the upper end of the small intestine. The narrow end of the pancreas, called the tail, extends to the left side of the body. The pancreas makes pancreatic juices and hormones, including insulin. Pancreatic juices are called enzymes that help digest food in the small intestine. Insulin controls the amount of sugar in the blood. Both hormones and enzymes are needed in order for the body to function right. As pancreatic juices are made, they flow into the main pancreatic duct, which connects the pancreas to the liver and the gallbladder. The common bile duct, which carries bile (a fluid that helps digest fat) connects to the small intestine near the stomach. More than 100 different types of cancer are known-and several types of cancer can develop in the pancreas. Cancer that starts in the pancreas is called pancreatic cancer. When pancreatic cancer spreads, it usually travels through the lymphatic system. The lymphatic system is made up of a network of thin tubes that branch like blood vessels into tissues all over the body. Cancer cells are carried through these vessels by lymph, a colorless watery fluid that carries cells that fights off infection. Along the network of lymphatic vessels are groups of small bean shaped organs that are called lymph nodes to find out if these lymph nodes are cancerous or not the surgeon will often remove the lymph nodes near the pancreas. Cancer cells can also be carried through the bloodstream to the liver, lungs, bone and to other organs. Pancreatic cancer that spreads to other organs is called metastatic pancreatic cancer.

SYMPTOMS

Pancreatic cancer has been called a "silent disease" because early cancer of the pancreas does not cause symptoms, if the tumor is blocking the common bile duct and bile cannot pass into the digestive system, the skin and whites of the eyes may become yellow, and the urine may become darker, this is called jaundice. As the cancer grows and spreads, pain is often developed in the upper abdomen and sometimes spreads to the back. The pain might become worse after the person eats or lie down. Pancreatic cancer can also cause nausea, loss of appetite, weight loss, weakness, dizziness, muscle spasms, diarrhea and chills. Cancer called islet cell cancer begins in the cells of the pancreas that produces insulin and other hormones, islet cells are called the islets of Langerhans, islet cell cancer can cause the pancreas to make too much insulin or hormones, these symptoms may be caused by other less serious problem, only your doctor can tell for sure.

DIAGNOSIS

The doctor will do a complete physical examination and ask about the patient personal, and family history. The doctor usually orders blood, urine and a stool test. The doctor may order a test called an upper GI series, and a barium swallow, for this test the patient drinks a barium solution before x-rays of the upper digestive system are taken. The barium shows an outline of the pancreas on the x-rays, also the doctor may order other test such as an angiogram which is a special xray of blood vessels. a CT scan may also be ordered, x-rays that gives detailed pictures of a cross section of the pancreas and a test called ERCP (endoscopic retrograde cholangial pancreatogram) a special test of the common bile duct. To perform this test, a long flexible tube which is a (endoscope) is passed down the patient's throat through the stomach and into the small intestine, a dye is injected into the common bile duct and x-rays pictures are taken. The doctor can also look through the endoscope and take samples of tissue. A biopsy is the only sure way the doctor can tell if cancer is present, the tissue samples ae examined under a microscope by a pathologist, a doctor who checks for cancer cells. Another way to remove tissue is with a long needle that is passed through the skin into the pancreas, this is called a needle biopsy, ultrasound or x-rays are used to guide the placement of the needle. another type of biopsy is a brush biopsy, this procedure is done during the ERCP the doctor inserts a very small brush through the endoscope into the bile duct to rub off cells to examine under a microscope, sometimes an operation called a laparotomy may be needed in order for the doctor to look at organs in the abdomen and can remove tissue. The laparotomy helps the doctor to determine the stage or extent of the cancer and also know what stage the cancer is in; this helps the doctor to plan treatment. Tissue samples that are obtained with one kind of biopsy may not give a clear diagnosis; the biopsy may need to be repeated using a different method.

TREATMENT

Treatment for pancreatic cancer depends on several factors such as the type, size and the extent of the tumor as well as the patient's age and general health. Cancer of the pancreas is curable only when it is found in its earliest stages before it has spread, otherwise it is very difficult to cure, symptoms can be relieved. Pancreatic cancer is treated with surgery, radiation therapy, or chemotherapy, sometimes several methods are used. Surgery may be done to remove all or part of the pancreas, sometimes it may be necessary to remove a portion of the stomach, the duodenum, and other nearby tissues, this is called a whipple procedure. In cases where the cancer in the pancreas cannot be removed, the doctor may be able to create a bypass around the common bile duct or the duodenum if either is blocked by the cancer. Surgery for cancer of the pancreas is a major operation, weight loss can be a serious problem for patients being treated for pancreatic cancer, and nutrition is an important part of the treatment plan.

CANCER OF THE STOMACH

The stomach is the chamber located between the end of the esophagus and the beginning of the small intestine. Digestion of food begins in the stomach. Cancer of the stomach like any other cancers is a disease of body cells. Cells are tiny structures that make up all parts of the body, the skin, the heart, lungs, bones and so on. Although cells of various organs differ in shape and function, all cells reproduce themselves by dividing. When cell division is not orderly, abnormal growth takes place. Masses of tissue called tumors build up tumors may be benign or malignant.

<u>SYMPTONS</u>

The first symptoms of stomach cancer are much like those of other digestive illnesses, persistent indigestion, a feeling of bloating discomfort after eating, slight nausea, loss of appetite, heartburn and sometimes mild stomach pain. Later symptoms may be blood in the stool (either red or black in color) vomiting, weight loss and pain. Anemia and lack of acid in the stomach are conditions often found in patients who have stomach cancer. Blood in the stool can be an indication of cancer in the gastrointestinal tract including the stomach. An x-ray of your stomach helps the doctor in making a diagnosis. For this exam you will be asked to drink a liquid containing barium sulfate, a substance that makes parts of your body more visible in x-ray pictures. Using an x-ray machine called a fluoroscope, the doctor can observe the flow of the barium sulfate into your stomach and can see the outline of your stomach from several different angles. The doctor can recognize an abnormality on the outline of the stomach seen with the fluoroscope. In some cases, the doctor may need to examine the stomach with an instrument passed through the mouth and esophagus. A sedative or anesthetic may be given before the exam so it is not so uncomfortable. One instrument that may be used is a flexible tube with a light and a series of mirrors that enables the doctor to see and take pictures of the inside of the stomach if a growth is detected, a small sample of tissue will be removed through the instrument. The removal and microscopic examination of a tissue is called a biopsy.

TREATMENT

Treatment is generally prompt removal of the tumor by surgery, this may require removing part of all of the stomach. if all the cancer present in the body cannot be removed by surgery, chemotherapy, treatment with anticancer drugs might be given. Anticancer drugs enter the bloodstream and circulate through the body to attack cancer in any location, because the drugs act on normal cells as well as cancerous cells. Radiation therapy plays a very limited role, in the treatment of stomach cancer, the reason is radiation doses are strong enough to destroy the cancer cells it could damage the surrounding tissue.

CANCER OF THE TESTIS

The testis or testicles are the primary male sex organ, which produces spermatozoa, the cells that fertilize the female egg during reproduction. The testes are oval shaped organs, suspended below the penis in a pouch of skin called the scrotum. Cancer of the testis is like other cancers, a disease of the body's cells, in the majority of cases only one testis is affected.

SYMPTONS

A small hard lump about the size of a pea in a testicle is the most common symptom of cancer of the testis. In the early stages of this disease, the lump is usually painless, giving no warning signs, other symptoms may include enlargement of a testicle, a heavy feeling in the testis, a sudden accumulation of fluid or blood in the scrotum. If the disease has spread, there may be swelling or tenderness in other parts of the body, such as the groin, breast or neck, these symptoms may not be due to cancer.

DIAGNOSIS

Most testicular cancers are discovered by men themselves, if you find a swelling, or hard lump or pain you need to see your doctor, a sample of tissue from the suspected area is examined under a microscope by a pathologist, a doctor who interprets and diagnoses the changes caused by disease in body tissue. In addition to plain x-rays of the chest and abdomen, special procedures such as intravenous pyelography and lymphangiography may show the spread of tumors that are otherwise not detectable. A total body scan or cat scan can also be used to check for spread of testicular cancer. When a diagnosis of cancer is confirmed its best to start treatment right away.

TREATMENT

Treatment of cancer of the testis always include surgical removal of the affected testis. If the cancer is localized, that may be the only treatment that is required, there is no fear that this will cause men to be impotent. One healthy testicle is fine for sexual function. If its suspected that cancer has spread to nearby lymph nodes, these also will be removed. Following surgery the patient may be treated with radiation therapy or chemotherapy a combination of both, radiation therapy uses x-rays, cobalt or other sources of ionizing radiation to destroy the cancer cells. Studies show that cancer of the testis occurs more frequently in young between the age of 20 to 40 the prime of life.

URINARY TRACT INFECTIONS

Infections of the urinary tract are the second most common type of infection in the body. After respiratory infections, the urinary tract, which consists of the kidneys, ureters, bladder and urethra is responsible for filtering and removing liquid waste from the body. The kidneys remove excess liquid and wastes from the blood the result is urine, The kidneys keep a stable balance of salts and other substances in the blood. A urinary tract infection is a bacterial infection that affects any part of the urinary tract. If a bladder infection is not treated, bacteria can travel higher up into the ureters and infect the kidneys, urinary tract infections are not only for women, men get them also. In men, enlargement of the prostate gland can put pressure on the urethra and the bladder opening, this prevents the bladder from emptying completely and may result in an infection. Other causes are waiting too long to urinate and holding your urine can cause the bladder which is a muscle to stretch beyond its capacity, when this happens it can weaken the bladder muscle, and prevent the bladder from emptying completely and increase the risk of infection. It is very important that anyone with a suspected urinary tract infections to see their doctor right away to avoid complication and potential kidney damage.

MY BIO

JACKIE YOUNG IS FOUNDER AND AUTHOR OF WHAT U NEED TO KNOW,AND WRITES HELFUL NEWSLETTERS MONTHLY ON YOU AND YOUR HEALTH.

www.ingramcontent.com/pod-product-compliance
Ingram Content Group UK Ltd.
Pitfield, Milton Keynes, MK11 3LW, UK
UKHW021028100325
455944UK00010B/483